STAGE 4 KIDNEY DISEASE DIET COOKBOOK FOR SENIORS

Easy and nutritious Recipes and Meal Plan Low in Sodium, Phosphorus and Potassium. Prevent and Manage CKD and acute renal failure.

Olivia Endwell

Copyright Statement:

Disclaimer:

The information provided in this book is for educational and informational purposes only. It is not intended as a substitute for professional medical advice, diagnosis, or treatment. Always seek the advice of your physician or other qualified health provider with any questions you may have regarding a medical condition. Never disregard professional medical advice or delay in seeking it because of something you have read in this book.

The author and publisher disclaim any liability arising directly or indirectly from the use of this book. The information provided is based on the author's best knowledge at the time of writing and is subject to change. The author and publisher do not guarantee the accuracy, completeness, or timeliness of the information presented in this book.

Individual results may vary, and the success of any dietary or lifestyle change depends on various factors, including but not limited to individual commitment and adherence. Before making significant changes to your diet or lifestyle, consult with a qualified healthcare professional

The views and opinions expressed in this book are those of the author and do not necessarily reflect the official policy or position of any other agency, organization, employer, or company.

TABLE OF CONTENTS

INTRODUCTION

Welcome to the culinary journey that awaits you in the "Stage 4 Kidney Disease Diet Cookbook for Seniors." In the pages that follow, we'll delve into the intricacies of understanding Stage 4 kidney disease and explore the profound importance of adopting a kidney-friendly diet, particularly tailored for seniors.

Imagine this cookbook as your friendly guide, navigating through the complexities of Stage 4 kidney disease. It's not just a collection of recipes; it's a companion for those navigating this stage of kidney health, especially in the golden years of life.

In the opening chapters, we'll unravel the mysteries of Stage 4 kidney disease, shedding light on what it means and how it affects individuals. This isn't just about medical jargon; it's about understanding your body and its unique needs during this phase.

As we journey together, we'll emphasize the crucial role that a kidney-friendly diet plays in the lives of seniors. It's not just about what you eat; it's about embracing a lifestyle that supports kidney health and overall well-being. We'll explore the nuances of nutrition, offering insights into how dietary choices can be a powerful tool in managing and even improving kidney function.

So, let's embark on this culinary adventure with a shared understanding of the challenges posed by Stage 4 kidney disease and the significance of adopting a diet that nurtures your kidneys.

Through delicious and carefully crafted recipes, we aim to make this journey not only manageable but also enjoyable. Get ready to savor the flavors of health and vitality!

THE BASICS OF STAGE 4 KIDNEY DISEASE

Overview of Kidney Function

In the intricate symphony of our bodies, the kidneys play a pivotal role, often working quietly behind the scenes. To truly understand Stage 4 Kidney Disease, one must first grasp the fundamentals of kidney function. Picture your kidneys as master chemists, filtering waste and excess fluids from the blood, while also regulating the body's electrolyte balance. These bean-shaped organs, each roughly the size of a fist, are the unsung heroes of our internal ecosystem.

Kidneys go beyond being mere filters; they contribute significantly to blood pressure regulation, red blood cell production, and the activation of vitamin D, crucial for bone health. As we delve into the complexities of kidney function, it becomes evident that their role is multi-faceted and indispensable. Understanding this foundation is key to comprehending the nuances of Stage 4 Kidney Disease.

Symptoms and Challenges in Stage 4

Now that we've established the importance of these renal maestros, let's explore what happens when they face the challenges of Stage 4 Kidney Disease. Symptoms in this stage can vary, and individuals may experience a range of issues such as fatigue, swelling, and changes in urination patterns. As the kidneys struggle to maintain their optimal function, waste products accumulate, leading to a cascade of complications.

One significant challenge is the impaired filtration of toxins, resulting in an increased concentration of waste in the bloodstream. This, in turn, can cause a domino effect on various bodily functions. Elevated blood pressure is a common companion in Stage 4, adding another layer of complexity to the management of the disease. The body's delicate balance of fluids and electrolytes is disrupted, leading to edema and fluid retention.

Challenges also extend to the cardiovascular system, with an increased risk of heart-related issues. Anemia often rears its head due to decreased production of erythropoietin, a hormone essential for red blood cell production. Bone health takes a hit as well, as the kidneys struggle to activate vitamin D, affecting calcium absorption and metabolism.

Navigating these symptoms and challenges requires a comprehensive approach that goes beyond medical interventions. It involves understanding the daily impact on an individual's life, addressing the physical and emotional toll, and finding ways to enhance overall well-being.

As we explore these intricacies, it's important to recognize that Stage 4 Kidney Disease is a journey, and each individual's experience is unique. By unraveling the intricacies of symptoms and challenges, we empower both individuals and caregivers to face this stage with knowledge, resilience, and a proactive mindset.

THE SENIOR PERSPECTIVE

Unique Considerations for Seniors with Kidney Disease

As we delve into the intricacies of Stage 4 Kidney Disease, it is imperative to consider the unique perspective that seniors bring to this health journey. The golden years often come with a tapestry of experiences, wisdom, and, inevitably, a collection of health concerns. When kidney disease becomes a companion in this stage of life, understanding the specific nuances and challenges becomes paramount.

Seniors with kidney disease encounter a distinctive set of considerations that stem from the aging process itself. One key aspect is the natural decline in kidney function that occurs with age, even without the presence of disease. This age-related decline can compound the challenges faced by those already navigating Stage 4 Kidney Disease. Recognizing and addressing these unique considerations is fundamental to providing tailored care and support.

Beyond the physiological changes, seniors may also contend with factors such as limited mobility, cognitive decline, and potential social isolation. These elements can significantly impact the management of kidney disease. For example, adherence to dietary restrictions and medication regimens may become more challenging, requiring a thoughtful and individualized approach to care.

Navigating the unique considerations for seniors involves a holistic perspective that goes beyond medical interventions. It requires a keen understanding of an individual's lifestyle, support systems, and personal goals. Recognizing the intersectionality of health and age is the first step towards creating a care plan that respects the individuality of each senior facing Stage 4 Kidney Disease.

Managing Kidney Disease Alongside Other Health Concerns

Seniors seldom navigate health challenges in isolation. Kidney disease often coexists with an array of other health concerns, creating a complex landscape that demands integrated and comprehensive management. Managing kidney disease alongside these coexisting conditions requires a delicate balance, acknowledging the interconnected nature of health in the senior years.

One common companion to kidney disease is hypertension. The interplay between kidney health and blood pressure regulation is intricate, and seniors with Stage 4 Kidney Disease often find themselves grappling with the dual challenge of managing both conditions. This necessitates not only careful medication management but also lifestyle adjustments that promote overall cardiovascular health.

Diabetes, another prevalent health concern in the senior population, can further complicate the picture. The intricate relationship between diabetes and kidney function adds layers to the management strategy. Seniors with both diabetes and Stage 4 Kidney Disease must navigate dietary restrictions, medication regimens, and lifestyle modifications with a nuanced understanding of how these conditions intersect.

Cognitive health is yet another dimension that cannot be overlooked. Seniors may face challenges in adhering to complex medication schedules or dietary restrictions due to cognitive decline. Tailoring care plans to accommodate these challenges is essential, emphasizing simplicity, clear communication, and support from caregivers.

Moreover, musculoskeletal issues, such as arthritis, can impact mobility and dietary choices. A holistic approach to care recognizes the interconnectedness of these health concerns and seeks to create a plan that addresses the unique combination of conditions each senior faces.

THE KIDNEY-FRIENDLY KITCHEN

Stocking a Kidney-Friendly Pantry

In the realm of managing Stage 4 Kidney Disease, the kitchen transforms into a sanctuary of healing. Building a kidney-friendly pantry is the first step on this culinary journey, laying the foundation for wholesome and nourishing meals that align with the unique dietary requirements of this stage. As we explore the elements to stock in a kidney-friendly pantry, the emphasis is not just on restriction but on the abundance of flavorful and health-promoting options.

1. Low-Potassium Ingredients: Potassium regulation is a crucial consideration in kidney-friendly cooking. Stock your pantry with low-potassium alternatives, such as apples, berries, cabbage, and green beans. These options allow for creativity in meal preparation while keeping potassium levels in check.

2. Phosphorus-Aware Choices: Phosphorus management is another key aspect. Opt for lower phosphorus options like rice, pasta, and bread. Incorporating grains and cereals with controlled phosphorus content provides a canvas for diverse and satisfying meals without compromising kidney health.

3. Low-Sodium Staples: Sodium restriction is a cornerstone of a kidney-friendly diet. Choose low-sodium alternatives for pantry essentials, including broths, canned vegetables, and sauces. Herbs and spices can step in as flavorful substitutes, enhancing dishes without the need for excess salt.

4. Heart-Healthy Oils: Fats are an essential part of any balanced diet, but choosing the right oils is crucial for kidney health. Opt for heart-healthy oils like olive oil or canola oil, rich in monounsaturated fats. These oils contribute to a favorable lipid profile without burdening the kidneys.

5. High-Quality Proteins: Protein remains a vital component, but the source matters. Stock your pantry with high-quality, low-phosphorus protein options, such as lean meats, poultry, and fish. Additionally, plant-based proteins like legumes and tofu offer versatile alternatives for those seeking non-animal protein sources.

6. Grains and Legumes: Whole grains and legumes provide a nutritious base for meals, offering fiber and essential nutrients. Brown rice, quinoa, and lentils are excellent choices, promoting satiety and contributing to overall well-being.

7. Fresh and Frozen Produce: Embrace the vibrancy of fresh and frozen fruits and vegetables. These nutrient-packed options form the backbone of a kidney-friendly diet, offering a spectrum of vitamins and minerals without the burden of excessive potassium or phosphorus.

Crafting a kidney-friendly pantry is not about restriction but about cultivating a selection of ingredients that nourish the body while respecting its unique needs. It's an invitation to explore the diverse and delicious world of wholesome foods, fostering a positive relationship with cooking and eating during Stage 4 Kidney Disease.

Essential Cooking Tools and Techniques

Equipping your kitchen with the right tools and mastering essential cooking techniques becomes an art form when managing Stage 4 Kidney Disease. This is not merely about culinary prowess but about embracing methods that enhance the nutritional value of meals while aligning with kidney health. Let's explore the essential cooking tools and techniques that transform the kitchen into a space of therapeutic gastronomy.

1. Precision Measuring Tools: Accurate measurement is crucial when managing nutrients like sodium, potassium, and phosphorus. Invest in precision measuring tools, including measuring cups and spoons, to ensure precise portions and adherence to dietary guidelines. This attention to detail is the cornerstone of crafting kidney-friendly meals.

2. Non-Stick Cookware: Non-stick cookware is a valuable addition to the kidney-friendly kitchen. It reduces the need for excessive oils and fats in cooking, promoting heart health while allowing for the creation of flavorful and satisfying dishes. It's a practical choice that aligns with the broader goal of maintaining a balanced and kidney-friendly diet.

3. Multi-Functional Appliances: Streamline your cooking process with multi-functional appliances like slow cookers, pressure cookers, and blenders. These tools not only save time but also offer versatile cooking methods. Slow cooking, for instance, allows flavors to meld without excessive salt, while blenders facilitate the creation of nutrient-rich soups and smoothies.

4. Fresh Herb Garden: Elevate the flavors of your dishes with a fresh herb garden. Growing herbs like basil, parsley, and chives at home not only adds an aromatic touch to your culinary creations but also provides a sodium-free way to enhance taste. Herbs become your allies in crafting kidney-friendly meals that are both delicious and nutritious.

5. Grilling and Roasting Techniques: Grilling and roasting are cooking techniques that bring out the natural flavors of ingredients without the need for excessive oils. These methods add depth and richness to dishes, offering a delightful culinary experience while adhering to kidney-friendly principles.

6. Batch Cooking and Portion Control: Embrace batch cooking as a time-saving strategy. Prepare kidney-friendly meals in larger quantities and portion them for future use. This approach not only streamlines meal preparation but also ensures that appropriate serving sizes are maintained, contributing to effective nutrient management.

7. Mindful Cooking Practices: Beyond the tools, mindful cooking practices play a significant role in kidney-friendly culinary endeavors. Pay attention to ingredient choices, experiment with new recipes, and savor the process of creating nourishing meals. Mindfulness in the kitchen fosters a positive relationship with food, promoting overall well-being.

NUTRITIONAL GUIDELINES FOR SENIORS WITH KIDNEY DISEASE

Understanding Nutrient Restrictions

In the intricate tapestry of managing Stage 4 Kidney Disease, understanding nutrient restrictions becomes a cornerstone for maintaining overall health. The delicate balance of nutrients, particularly sodium, potassium, and phosphorus, plays a pivotal role in mitigating the progression of kidney disease and alleviating associated symptoms. Let's unravel the nuances of these nutrient restrictions, exploring the impact they have on the body and how a tailored approach to diet can pave the way for enhanced well-being.

1. Sodium Management: Sodium, a ubiquitous component in many diets, takes center stage in kidney health. Seniors with Stage 4 Kidney Disease often face challenges related to fluid retention and elevated blood pressure, making sodium restriction imperative. Understanding hidden sources of sodium in processed foods and adopting mindful cooking practices that limit salt usage are crucial steps. Additionally, incorporating herbs and spices to enhance flavor without relying on sodium becomes a culinary art in the journey towards a kidney-friendly diet.

2. Potassium Awareness: Potassium regulation is another vital aspect of nutrient management for seniors with kidney disease. While potassium is an essential nutrient for various bodily functions, impaired kidney function can lead to potassium buildup, posing risks to heart health. Seniors must navigate a potassium-conscious diet, emphasizing low-potassium choices such as apples, berries, and cauliflower. This not only ensures proper nutrient intake but also reduces the burden on the kidneys, contributing to a balanced and supportive dietary approach.

3. Phosphorus Monitoring: Phosphorus, a mineral crucial for bone health, requires careful monitoring in the context of kidney disease. Elevated phosphorus levels can lead to complications such as bone and cardiovascular issues. Seniors must be mindful of phosphorus-rich foods, including dairy products, nuts, and seeds. Strategic choices involving lower phosphorus alternatives like rice and pasta contribute to a well-rounded diet that aligns with the nutritional guidelines for Stage 4 Kidney Disease.

Understanding nutrient restrictions is not about deprivation but about making informed choices that nourish the body while respecting its unique needs. It involves a culinary dance of creativity and mindfulness, where each meal becomes an opportunity to support kidney health and overall wellness.

Tips for Maintaining a Balanced Diet

Navigating the realm of nutritional guidelines for seniors with kidney disease extends beyond understanding restrictions. It involves embracing a holistic approach that fosters a balanced and nourishing diet, promoting overall well-being. Let's delve into practical tips that empower seniors to maintain a balanced diet, incorporating a spectrum of nutrients while respecting the unique requirements of Stage 4 Kidney Disease.

1. Individualized Meal Planning: Recognizing the individuality of each senior is paramount in maintaining a balanced diet. Tailoring meal plans to accommodate personal preferences, cultural backgrounds, and dietary tolerances ensures that adherence to nutritional guidelines becomes a sustainable and enjoyable endeavor. Individualized meal planning considers not only nutrient restrictions but also the diverse tastes and lifestyles of seniors, fostering a positive relationship with food.

2. Regular Monitoring and Consultation: Regular monitoring of kidney function and consultation with healthcare professionals form the backbone of a balanced diet for seniors with kidney disease. Periodic assessments of blood tests and discussions with healthcare providers allow for adjustments to dietary recommendations based on individual health status. This dynamic approach ensures that nutritional guidelines remain aligned with evolving health needs, promoting optimal kidney function and overall wellness.

3. Hydration as a Priority: Adequate hydration is a cornerstone of kidney health. Seniors must prioritize water intake to support proper kidney function and flush out toxins. However, it's essential to strike a balance, as excessive fluid intake can strain the kidneys. Consultation with healthcare professionals helps determine an individualized hydration plan, considering factors such as urine output, medications, and existing health conditions.

4. Mindful Portion Control: Portion control is a practical strategy in maintaining a balanced diet. Seniors with kidney disease can benefit from mindful portioning, which not only helps manage nutrient intake but also supports weight management. Balancing portion sizes with nutrient content allows for the enjoyment of a variety of foods while adhering to dietary guidelines.

5. Focus on Nutrient-Dense Foods: Emphasizing nutrient-dense foods is a key principle in crafting a balanced diet. Seniors should prioritize whole, unprocessed foods that pack a nutritional punch without burdening the kidneys. Incorporating a rainbow of fruits and vegetables, lean proteins, and whole grains ensures that each bite contributes to overall health while aligning with the nutritional guidelines for Stage 4 Kidney Disease.

6. Regular Physical Activity: Physical activity complements a balanced diet in promoting overall wellness. Seniors should engage in regular, moderate exercise to support cardiovascular health, weight management, and mental well-being. Exercise also contributes to better blood pressure control, a crucial factor in the management of kidney disease.

BREAKFAST RECIPES

1. Quinoa Breakfast Bowl

Prep Time: 10 minutes

Cooking Time: 15 minutes

Serving Size: 1

Ingredients:

- 1/2 cup quinoa, rinsed

- 1 cup almond milk

- 1/2 cup blueberries

- 1 tablespoon chopped walnuts

- 1 teaspoon honey

Instructions:

1. In a saucepan, combine quinoa and almond milk. Bring to a boil, then reduce heat, cover, and simmer for 15 minutes.

2. Fluff quinoa with a fork and transfer to a bowl.

3. Top with blueberries, chopped walnuts, and drizzle with honey.

4. Serve warm.

Nutritional Information:

- Calories: 350

- Protein: 10g

- Fiber: 7g

- Potassium: 300mg

- Phosphorus: 150mg

2. Spinach and Feta Omelette

Prep Time: 5 minutes

Cooking Time: 10 minutes

Serving Size: 1

Ingredients:

- 2 eggs, beaten

- 1/4 cup chopped spinach

- 2 tablespoons crumbled feta cheese

- Salt and pepper to taste

- 1 teaspoon olive oil

Instructions:

1. Heat olive oil in a non-stick skillet over medium heat.

2. Add chopped spinach and sauté until wilted.

3. Pour beaten eggs over spinach, sprinkle with feta, salt, and pepper.

4. Cook until eggs are set, then fold in half.

5. Serve hot.

Nutritional Information:

- Calories: 280

- Protein: 18g

- Fiber: 2g

- Potassium: 200mg

- Phosphorus: 180mg

3. Banana Walnut Pancakes

Prep Time: 15 minutes

Cooking Time: 10 minutes

Serving Size: 2 pancakes

Ingredients:

- 1/2 cup oat flour

- 1/2 teaspoon baking powder

- 1/4 teaspoon cinnamon

- 1/2 ripe banana, mashed

- 1/4 cup chopped walnuts

- 1/2 cup almond milk

Instructions:

1. In a bowl, mix oat flour, baking powder, and cinnamon.

2. Add mashed banana, chopped walnuts, and almond milk. Stir until well combined.

3. Heat a griddle or non-stick pan over medium heat.

4. Pour 1/4 cup of batter for each pancake.

5. Cook until bubbles form, then flip and cook the other side.

6. Serve with a dollop of Greek yogurt if desired.

Nutritional Information:

- Calories: 320

- Protein: 9g

- Fiber: 5g

- Potassium: 250mg

- Phosphorus: 200mg

4. Berry and Chia Seed Parfait

Prep Time: 5 minutes (plus overnight soaking)

Cooking Time: 0 minutes

Serving Size: 1

Ingredients:

- 2 tablespoons chia seeds

- 1/2 cup almond milk

- 1/2 cup mixed berries (strawberries, blueberries, raspberries)

- 1/4 cup granola

Instructions:

1. Mix chia seeds with almond milk, stir well, and refrigerate overnight.

2. In the morning, layer chia pudding with mixed berries in a glass.

3. Top with granola just before serving.

Nutritional Information:

- Calories: 280

- Protein: 7g

- Fiber: 12g

- Potassium: 180mg

- Phosphorus: 120mg

5. Sweet Potato Breakfast Hash

Prep Time: 10 minutes

Cooking Time: 20 minutes

Serving Size: 1

Ingredients:

- 1/2 cup diced sweet potatoes

- 1/4 cup diced bell peppers

- 1/4 cup diced onions

- 1 tablespoon olive oil

- 1/4 teaspoon smoked paprika

- Salt and pepper to taste

Instructions:

1. Heat olive oil in a skillet over medium heat.

2. Add sweet potatoes, bell peppers, and onions.

3. Sprinkle with smoked paprika, salt, and pepper.

4. Cook until sweet potatoes are tender and lightly browned.

5. Serve hot.

Nutritional Information:

- Calories: 260

- Protein: 3g

- Fiber: 5g

- Potassium: 220mg

- Phosphorus: 80mg

6. Avocado Toast with Smoked Salmon

Prep Time: 5 minutes

Cooking Time: 0 minutes

Serving Size: 1

Ingredients:

- 1 slice whole-grain bread

- 1/2 ripe avocado, mashed

- 2 ounces smoked salmon

- Lemon juice, salt, and pepper to taste

Instructions:

1. Toast the whole-grain bread slice.

2. Spread mashed avocado on the toast.

3. Top with smoked salmon.

4. Squeeze lemon juice over the top and season with salt and pepper.

5. Serve immediately.

Nutritional Information:

- Calories: 300

- Protein: 15g

- Fiber: 8g

- Potassium: 400mg

- Phosphorus: 150mg

7. Greek Yogurt Parfait

Prep Time: 5 minutes

Cooking Time: 0 minutes

Serving Size: 1

Ingredients:

- 1/2 cup Greek yogurt

- 1/4 cup granola

- 1/4 cup mixed berries (strawberries, blueberries, raspberries)

- 1 tablespoon honey

Instructions:

1. In a glass or bowl, layer Greek yogurt, granola, and mixed berries.

2. Drizzle honey over the top.

3. Repeat for additional layers if desired.

4. Serve chilled.

Nutritional Information:

- Calories: 280

- Protein: 18g

- Fiber: 4g

- Potassium: 220mg

- Phosphorus: 150mg

8. Veggie Breakfast Burrito

Prep Time: 15 minutes

Cooking Time: 10 minutes

Serving Size: 1

Ingredients:

- 1 whole-grain tortilla

- 2 eggs, scrambled

- 1/4 cup black beans, drained and rinsed

- 2 tablespoons diced tomatoes

- 2 tablespoons diced bell peppers

- 1 tablespoon shredded low-phosphorus cheese

- Salsa for serving

Instructions:

1. Heat the tortilla in a dry skillet or microwave until warm.

2. In a separate skillet, scramble the eggs.

3. Assemble the burrito by layering eggs, black beans,
   tomatoes, bell peppers, and cheese on the tortilla.

4. Roll it up and serve with salsa on the side.

Nutritional Information:

- Calories: 340

- Protein: 20g

- Fiber: 8g

- Potassium: 280mg

- Phosphorus: 200mg

9. Overnight Oats with Almond Butter

Prep Time: 5 minutes (plus overnight soaking)

Cooking Time: 0 minutes

Serving Size: 1

Ingredients:

- 1/2 cup rolled oats

- 1/2 cup almond milk

- 1 tablespoon almond butter

- 1/2 banana, sliced

- 1 teaspoon chia seeds

Instructions:

1. In a jar, combine rolled oats, almond milk, almond butter, banana slices, and chia seeds.

2. Stir well, cover, and refrigerate overnight.

3. In the morning, give it a good stir and enjoy.

Nutritional Information:

- Calories: 350

- Protein: 10g

- Fiber: 8g

- Potassium: 230mg

- Phosphorus: 180mg

10. Cottage Cheese and Pineapple Bowl

Prep Time: 5 minutes

Cooking Time: 0 minutes

Serving Size: 1

Ingredients:

- 1/2 cup low-fat cottage cheese

- 1/2 cup fresh pineapple chunks

- 1 tablespoon chopped mint (optional)

- 1 tablespoon sunflower seeds

Instructions:

1. In a bowl, combine cottage cheese and fresh pineapple chunks.

2. Sprinkle with chopped mint if desired.

3. Top with sunflower seeds.

4. Serve chilled.

Nutritional Information:

- Calories: 280

- Protein: 18g

- Fiber: 3g

- Potassium: 220mg

- Phosphorus: 180mg

11. Blueberry Almond Smoothie Bowl

Prep Time: 5 minutes

Cooking Time: 0 minutes

Serving Size: 1

Ingredients:

- 1/2 cup frozen blueberries

- 1/2 banana

- 1/2 cup almond milk

- 1 tablespoon almond butter

- 1 tablespoon chia seeds

- 1 tablespoon sliced almonds

Instructions:

1. Blend frozen blueberries, banana, almond milk, and almond butter until smooth.

2. Pour into a bowl.

3. Top with chia seeds and sliced almonds.

4. Serve immediately.

Nutritional Information:

- Calories: 320

- Protein: 9g

- Fiber: 10g

- Potassium: 250mg

- Phosphorus: 200mg

12. Smashed Avocado and Tomato Toast

Prep Time: 5 minutes

Cooking Time: 0 minutes

Serving Size: 1

Ingredients:

- 1 slice whole-grain bread

- 1/2 ripe avocado, smashed

- 1/2 cup cherry tomatoes, halved

- Fresh basil leaves

- Balsamic glaze for drizzling

Instructions:

1. Toast the whole-grain bread slice.

2. Spread smashed avocado on the toast.

3. Arrange cherry tomato halves on top.

4. Garnish with fresh basil leaves.

5. Drizzle with balsamic glaze.

6. Serve immediately.

Nutritional Information:

- Calories: 290

- Protein: 8g

- Fiber: 7g

- Potassium: 320mg

- Phosphorus: 180mg

13. Buckwheat and Berry Breakfast Bowl

Prep Time: 10 minutes

Cooking Time: 15 minutes

Serving Size: 1

Ingredients:

- 1/2 cup cooked buckwheat groats

- 1/2 cup mixed berries (strawberries, blueberries, raspberries)

- 1 tablespoon chopped pistachios

- 1 tablespoon honey

- 1/2 teaspoon vanilla extract

Instructions:

1. Cook buckwheat groats according to package instructions.

2. In a bowl, combine cooked buckwheat, mixed berries, chopped pistachios, honey, and vanilla extract.

3. Mix well and serve.

Nutritional Information:

- Calories: 300

- Protein: 8g

- Fiber: 6g

- Potassium: 200mg

- Phosphorus: 150mg

14. Rice Cake with Almond Cream Cheese and Berries

Prep Time: 5 minutes

Cooking Time: 0 minutes

Serving Size: 1

Ingredients:

- 1 rice cake

- 2 tablespoons almond cream cheese

- 1/4 cup mixed berries (strawberries, blueberries, raspberries)

- 1 teaspoon chia seeds

Instructions:

1. Spread almond cream cheese on the rice cake.

2. Top with mixed berries.

3. Sprinkle with chia seeds.

4. Serve immediately.

Nutritional Information:

- Calories: 220

- Protein: 6g

- Fiber: 4g

- Potassium: 180mg

- Phosphorus: 120mg

15. Muesli with Yogurt and Mango

Prep Time: 5 minutes

Cooking Time: 0 minutes

Serving Size: 1

Ingredients:

- 1/2 cup low-fat plain yogurt

- 1/4 cup muesli

- 1/2 mango, diced

- 1 tablespoon pumpkin seeds

Instructions:

1. In a bowl, layer low-fat plain yogurt with muesli.

2. Top with diced mango and pumpkin seeds.

3. Serve chilled.

Nutritional Information:

- Calories: 270

- Protein: 9g

- Fiber: 4g

- Potassium: 280mg

- Phosphorus: 150mg

16. Apple Cinnamon Chia Pudding

Prep Time: 10 minutes (plus overnight soaking)

Cooking Time: 0 minutes

Serving Size: 1

Ingredients:

- 2 tablespoons chia seeds

- 1/2 cup almond milk

- 1/2 apple, diced

- 1/4 teaspoon cinnamon

- 1 tablespoon chopped pecans

Instructions:

1. Mix chia seeds with almond milk, stir well, and refrigerate overnight.

2. In the morning, layer chia pudding with diced apple in a glass.

3. Sprinkle with cinnamon and chopped pecans.

4. Serve chilled.

Nutritional Information:

- Calories: 280

- Protein: 7g

- Fiber: 10g

- Potassium: 220mg

- Phosphorus: 180mg

17. Egg and Asparagus Breakfast Wrap

Prep Time: 10 minutes

Cooking Time: 10 minutes

Serving Size: 1

Ingredients:

- 1 whole-grain tortilla

- 2 eggs, scrambled

- 4 asparagus spears, blanched

- 1 tablespoon grated low-phosphorus cheese

- Salt and pepper to taste

Instructions:

1. Heat the whole-grain tortilla in a dry skillet or microwave until warm.

2. Scramble the eggs and cook until just set.

3. Lay blanched asparagus spears on the tortilla.

4. Top with scrambled eggs, grated cheese, salt, and pepper.

5. Roll it up and serve.

Nutritional Information:

- Calories: 320

- Protein: 18g

- Fiber: 6g

- Potassium: 280mg

- Phosphorus: 200mg

18. Buckwheat Pancakes with Berry Compote

Prep Time: 15 minutes

Cooking Time: 10 minutes

Serving Size: 2 pancakes

Ingredients:

- 1/2 cup buckwheat flour

- 1/2 teaspoon baking powder

- 1/4 teaspoon cinnamon

- 1/2 cup almond milk

- 1/2 cup mixed berries (strawberries, blueberries, raspberries)

- 1 tablespoon maple syrup

Instructions:

1. In a bowl, whisk together buckwheat flour, baking powder, and cinnamon.

2. Add almond milk and mix until smooth.

3. Heat a griddle or non-stick pan over medium heat.

4. Pour 1/4 cup of batter for each pancake.

5. Cook until bubbles form, then flip and cook the other side.

6. In a separate saucepan, heat mixed berries and maple syrup to create a compote.

7. Top pancakes with berry compote and serve.

Nutritional Information:

- Calories: 340

- Protein: 10g

- Fiber: 8g

- Potassium: 250mg

- Phosphorus: 180mg

19. Tomato Basil Frittata

Prep Time: 10 minutes

Cooking Time: 20 minutes

Serving Size: 2

Ingredients:

- 4 eggs, beaten

- 1/2 cup cherry tomatoes, halved

- 2 tablespoons chopped fresh basil

- 1/4 cup grated low-phosphorus cheese

- Salt and pepper to taste

- 1 teaspoon olive oil

Instructions:

1. Preheat the oven to 350°F (180°C).

2. In a bowl, whisk together beaten eggs, cherry tomatoes, chopped basil, grated cheese, salt, and pepper.

3. Heat olive oil in an oven-safe skillet over medium heat.

4. Pour the egg mixture into the skillet and cook for 2-3 minutes.

5. Transfer the skillet to the preheated oven and bake for 15-18 minutes or until the frittata is set.

6. Slice and serve.

Nutritional Information:

- Calories: 320

- Protein: 18g

- Fiber: 2g

- Potassium: 300mg

- Phosphorus: 200mg

20. Almond Flour Waffles with Berries

Prep Time: 10 minutes

Cooking Time: 15 minutes

Serving Size: 2 waffles

Ingredients:

- 1 cup almond flour

- 1/2 teaspoon baking powder

- 2 eggs

- 1/2 cup almond milk

- 1/2 teaspoon vanilla extract

- 1/2 cup mixed berries (strawberries, blueberries, raspberries)

- 1 tablespoon Greek yogurt (optional)

Instructions:

1. In a bowl, combine almond flour and baking powder.

2. Add eggs, almond milk, and vanilla extract. Mix until smooth.

3. Preheat a waffle iron and grease with cooking spray.

4. Pour batter onto the hot waffle iron and cook according to the manufacturer's instructions.

5. Top waffles with mixed berries and a dollop of Greek yogurt if desired.

6. Serve warm.

Nutritional Information:

- Calories: 350

- Protein: 15g

- Fiber: 6g

- Potassium: 230mg

- Phosphorus: 180mg

LUNCH RECIPES

1. Lemon Herb Grilled Chicken

Prep Time: 15 minutes

Cooking Time: 20 minutes

Serving Size: 1

Ingredients:

- 4 oz boneless, skinless chicken breast

- 1 tablespoon olive oil

- 1 tablespoon lemon juice

- 1 teaspoon dried oregano

- 1 teaspoon dried thyme

- Salt and pepper to taste

Instructions:

1. Preheat the grill to medium-high heat.

2. In a bowl, mix olive oil, lemon juice, oregano, thyme, salt, and pepper.

3. Marinate chicken in the mixture for 10 minutes.

4. Grill chicken for 8-10 minutes per side or until fully cooked.

5. Serve hot.

Nutritional Information:

- Calories: 280

- Protein: 30g

- Fiber: 0g

- Potassium: 320mg

- Phosphorus: 200mg

2. Quinoa and Vegetable Stir-Fry

Prep Time: 10 minutes

Cooking Time: 15 minutes

Serving Size: 1

Ingredients:

- 1/2 cup quinoa, cooked

- 1/2 cup broccoli florets

- 1/2 cup bell peppers, sliced

- 1/2 cup snap peas

- 1 tablespoon low-sodium soy sauce

- 1 teaspoon sesame oil

Instructions:

1. In a wok or skillet, heat sesame oil over medium-high heat.

2. Add broccoli, bell peppers, and snap peas. Stir-fry for 5-7 minutes.

3. Add cooked quinoa and soy sauce. Mix well.

4. Cook for an additional 3-5 minutes.

5. Serve warm.

Nutritional Information:

- Calories: 320

- Protein: 12g

- Fiber: 8g

- Potassium: 280mg

- Phosphorus: 150mg

3. Baked Salmon with Dill Sauce

Prep Time: 10 minutes

Cooking Time: 15 minutes

Serving Size: 1

Ingredients:

- 4 oz salmon fillet

- 1 tablespoon olive oil

- 1 teaspoon dried dill

- Salt and pepper to taste

- 2 tablespoons plain Greek yogurt

- 1 teaspoon lemon juice

Instructions:

1. Preheat the oven to 400°F (200°C).

2. Place salmon on a baking sheet and drizzle with olive oil.

3. Sprinkle with dried dill, salt, and pepper.

4. Bake for 12-15 minutes or until salmon is cooked through.

5. In a small bowl, mix Greek yogurt and lemon juice for the sauce.

6. Serve salmon with dill sauce.

Nutritional Information:

- Calories: 320

- Protein: 25g

- Fiber: 0g

- Potassium: 400mg

- Phosphorus: 180mg

4. Turkey and Vegetable Skewers

Prep Time: 20 minutes

Cooking Time: 15 minutes

Serving Size: 1

Ingredients:

- 4 oz turkey breast, cut into cubes

- 1/2 zucchini, sliced

- 1/2 red onion, sliced

- 1/2 red bell pepper, diced

- 1 tablespoon olive oil

- 1 teaspoon dried rosemary

- Salt and pepper to taste

Instructions:

1. Preheat the grill or grill pan.

2. Thread turkey, zucchini, red onion, and red bell pepper onto skewers.

3. In a bowl, mix olive oil, dried rosemary, salt, and pepper.

4. Brush skewers with the olive oil mixture.

5. Grill for 10-12 minutes, turning occasionally, until turkey is cooked.

6. Serve hot.

Nutritional Information:

- Calories: 290

- Protein: 30g

- Fiber: 4g

- Potassium: 350mg

- Phosphorus: 220mg

5. Eggplant and Tomato Stew

Prep Time: 15 minutes

Cooking Time: 25 minutes

Serving Size: 1

Ingredients:

- 1 small eggplant, diced

- 1 cup cherry tomatoes, halved

- 1/2 cup red bell pepper, chopped

- 1/4 cup red onion, diced

- 1 tablespoon olive oil

- 1 teaspoon dried basil

- Salt and pepper to taste

Instructions:

1. Heat olive oil in a skillet over medium heat.

2. Add eggplant, cherry tomatoes, red bell pepper, and red onion.

3. Cook for 20-25 minutes, stirring occasionally.

4. Season with dried basil, salt, and pepper.

5. Serve as a stew or over cooked quinoa.

Nutritional Information:

- Calories: 250

- Protein: 5g

- Fiber: 8g

- Potassium: 300mg

- Phosphorus: 120mg

6. Lentil and Vegetable Soup

Prep Time: 15 minutes

Cooking Time: 30 minutes

Serving Size: 1

Ingredients:

- 1/2 cup dried green lentils, rinsed

- 1 carrot, diced

- 1 celery stalk, diced

- 1/2 cup onion, chopped

- 2 cups low-sodium vegetable broth

- 1 teaspoon olive oil

- 1 teaspoon dried thyme

- Salt and pepper to taste

Instructions:

1. In a pot, heat olive oil over medium heat.

2. Add onion, carrot, and celery. Sauté for 5 minutes.

3. Add lentils, vegetable broth, dried thyme, salt, and pepper.

4. Bring to a boil, then reduce heat and simmer for 25-30 minutes.

5. Serve hot.

Nutritional Information:

- Calories: 280

- Protein: 18g

- Fiber: 10g

- Potassium: 400mg

- Phosphorus: 200mg

7. Shrimp and Asparagus Stir-Fry

Prep Time: 10 minutes

Cooking Time: 10 minutes

Serving Size: 1

Ingredients:

- 4 oz shrimp, peeled and deveined

- 1/2 bunch asparagus, trimmed and cut into 2-inch pieces

- 1 tablespoon low-sodium soy sauce

- 1 tablespoon sesame oil

- 1 teaspoon ginger, minced

- 1 teaspoon garlic, minced

Instructions:

1. In a wok or skillet, heat sesame oil over medium-high heat.

2. Add shrimp, asparagus, ginger, and garlic. Stir-fry for 5-7 minutes.

3. Add soy sauce and continue cooking for an additional 2-3 minutes.

4. Serve over cooked brown rice or quinoa.

Nutritional Information:

- Calories: 290

- Protein: 25g

- Fiber: 5g

- Potassium: 350mg

- Phosphorus: 200mg

8. Chicken and Vegetable Wrap

Prep Time: 15 minutes

Cooking Time: 10 minutes

Serving Size: 1

Ingredients:

- 4 oz grilled chicken breast, sliced

- 1 whole-grain tortilla

- 1/4 cup hummus

- 1/2 cup mixed greens

- 1/4 cup cucumber, sliced

- 1 tablespoon feta cheese, crumbled

Instructions:

1. Spread hummus on the whole-grain tortilla.

2. Layer with grilled chicken, mixed greens, cucumber, and feta cheese.

3. Roll up the tortilla and secure with a toothpick.

4. Slice in half and serve.

Nutritional Information:

- Calories: 330

- Protein: 30g

- Fiber: 8g

- Potassium: 380mg

- Phosphorus: 220mg

9. Spinach and Mushroom Frittata

Prep Time: 10 minutes

Cooking Time: 20 minutes

Serving Size: 2

Ingredients:

- 4 eggs, beaten

- 1 cup spinach, chopped

- 1/2 cup mushrooms, sliced

- 1/4 cup onion, diced

- 1 tablespoon olive oil

- Salt and pepper to taste

Instructions:

1. Preheat the oven to 350°F (180°C).

2. In an oven-safe skillet, heat olive oil over medium heat.

3. Sauté mushrooms and onion until softened.

4. Add chopped spinach and cook until wilted.

5. Pour beaten eggs over the vegetables. Season with salt and pepper.

6. Cook on the stovetop for 2-3 minutes, then transfer to the oven and bake for 15-18 minutes or until set.

7. Slice and serve.

Nutritional Information:

- Calories: 310

- Protein: 18g

- Fiber: 3g

- Potassium: 300mg

- Phosphorus: 180mg

10. Tofu and Vegetable Stir-Fry

Prep Time: 15 minutes

Cooking Time: 15 minutes

Serving Size: 1

Ingredients:

- 1/2 cup firm tofu, cubed

- 1/2 cup broccoli florets

- 1/2 cup snow peas

- 1/2 cup carrots, sliced

- 1 tablespoon low-sodium soy sauce

- 1 teaspoon sesame oil

- 1 teaspoon garlic, minced

Instructions:

1. In a wok or skillet, heat sesame oil over medium-high heat.

2. Add tofu, broccoli, snow peas, and carrots. Stir-fry for 8-10 minutes.

3. Add minced garlic and soy sauce. Continue cooking for an additional 2-3 minutes.

4. Serve over cooked brown rice or quinoa.

Nutritional Information:

- Calories: 270

- Protein: 15g

- Fiber: 7g

- Potassium: 320mg

- Phosphorus: 180mg

11. Avocado and Chickpea Salad

Prep Time: 10 minutes

Cooking Time: 0 minutes

Serving Size: 1

Ingredients:

- 1/2 avocado, diced

- 1/2 cup canned chickpeas, drained and rinsed

- 1/4 cup cherry tomatoes, halved

- 1/4 cup cucumber, diced

- 1 tablespoon olive oil

- 1 tablespoon balsamic vinegar

- Salt and pepper to taste

Instructions:

1. In a bowl, combine diced avocado, chickpeas, cherry tomatoes, and cucumber.

2. Drizzle with olive oil and balsamic vinegar. Toss gently.

3. Season with salt and pepper.

4. Serve chilled.

Nutritional Information:

- Calories: 320

- Protein: 8g

- Fiber: 10g

- Potassium: 400mg

- Phosphorus: 200mg

12. Mediterranean Turkey Burger

Prep Time: 15 minutes

Cooking Time: 15 minutes

Serving Size: 1

Ingredients:

- 4 oz ground turkey

- 1/4 cup feta cheese, crumbled

- 1/4 cup Kalamata olives, chopped

- 1 teaspoon dried oregano

- 1 whole-grain burger bun

- Lettuce, tomato, and red onion for garnish

Instructions:

1. In a bowl, mix ground turkey, feta cheese, chopped olives, and dried oregano.

2. Form into a patty and grill for 7-8 minutes per side or until fully cooked.

3. Toast the burger bun on the grill for 1-2 minutes.

4. Assemble the burger with lettuce, tomato, red onion, and the turkey patty.

5. Serve hot.

Nutritional Information:

- Calories: 350

- Protein: 25g

- Fiber: 5g

- Potassium: 320mg

- Phosphorus: 200mg

13. Caprese Salad with Grilled Chicken

Prep Time: 10 minutes

Cooking Time: 15 minutes

Serving Size: 1

Ingredients:

- 4 oz grilled chicken breast, sliced

- 1 cup cherry tomatoes, halved

- 1/2 cup fresh mozzarella, diced

- Fresh basil leaves

- 1 tablespoon balsamic glaze

- Salt and pepper to taste

Instructions:

1. Arrange grilled chicken, cherry tomatoes, and fresh mozzarella on a plate.

2. Garnish with fresh basil leaves.

3. Drizzle with balsamic glaze and season with salt and pepper.

4. Serve at room temperature.

Nutritional Information:

- Calories: 320

- Protein: 30g

- Fiber: 2g

- Potassium: 380mg

- Phosphorus: 220mg

14. Cauliflower and Chickpea Curry

Prep Time: 15 minutes

Cooking Time: 25 minutes

Serving Size: 1

Ingredients:

- 1 cup cauliflower florets

- 1/2 cup canned chickpeas, drained and rinsed

- 1/2 cup tomatoes, diced

- 1/4 cup onion, chopped

- 1 tablespoon coconut oil

- 1 teaspoon curry powder

- 1/2 cup low-sodium vegetable broth

Instructions:

1. In a pot, heat coconut oil over medium heat.

2. Add onion and sauté until translucent.

3. Stir in curry powder and cook for 1-2 minutes.

4. Add cauliflower, chickpeas, tomatoes, and vegetable broth.

5. Simmer for 20-25 minutes or until cauliflower is tender.

6. Serve over brown rice.

Nutritional Information:

- Calories: 290

- Protein: 12g

- Fiber: 8g

- Potassium: 350mg

- Phosphorus: 180mg

15. Turkey and Sweet Potato Hash

Prep Time: 15 minutes

Cooking Time: 20 minutes

Serving Size: 1

Ingredients:

- 4 oz ground turkey

- 1/2 cup sweet potato, diced

- 1/4 cup bell peppers, diced

- 1/4 cup onion, diced

- 1 tablespoon olive oil

- 1 teaspoon smoked paprika

- Salt and pepper to taste

Instructions:

1. In a skillet, heat olive oil over medium heat.

2. Add ground turkey, sweet potato, bell peppers, and onion.

3. Cook until turkey is browned and sweet potatoes are tender.

4. Season with smoked paprika, salt, and pepper.

5. Serve hot.

Nutritional Information:

- Calories: 310

- Protein: 20g

- Fiber: 5g

- Potassium: 380mg

- Phosphorus: 200mg

16. Broccoli and Chicken Alfredo Pasta

Prep Time: 15 minutes

Cooking Time: 20 minutes

Serving Size: 1

Ingredients:

- 2 oz whole-grain fettuccine pasta

- 4 oz grilled chicken breast, sliced

- 1 cup broccoli florets

- 1/2 cup low-fat Alfredo sauce

- 1 tablespoon Parmesan cheese, grated

Instructions:

1. Cook pasta according to package instructions.

2. In a pot, steam broccoli until tender.

3. Heat Alfredo sauce in a skillet over low heat.

4. Add sliced grilled chicken to the sauce and stir until heated through.

5. Combine cooked pasta, broccoli, and Alfredo chicken.

6. Sprinkle with Parmesan cheese and serve.

Nutritional Information:

- Calories: 340

- Protein: 30g

- Fiber: 6g

- Potassium: 400mg

- Phosphorus: 220mg

17. Spaghetti Squash with Marinara Sauce

Prep Time: 15 minutes

Cooking Time: 45 minutes

Serving Size: 1

Ingredients:

- 1/2 medium spaghetti squash

- 1/2 cup marinara sauce (low-sodium)

- 1/4 cup grated low-fat mozzarella cheese

- Fresh basil leaves for garnish

Instructions:

1. Preheat the oven to 375°F (190°C).

2. Cut spaghetti squash in half and scoop out the seeds.

3. Place the squash, cut side down, on a baking sheet.

4. Bake for 40-45 minutes or until the flesh is tender.

5. Scrape the squash with a fork to create "spaghetti" strands.

6. Top with marinara sauce, mozzarella cheese, and fresh basil leaves.

7. Bake for an additional 5 minutes or until cheese is melted.

8. Serve warm.

Nutritional Information:

- Calories: 280

- Protein: 8g

- Fiber: 7g

- Potassium: 350mg

- Phosphorus: 180mg

18. Seared Tuna Salad with Sesame Dressing

Prep Time: 10 minutes

Cooking Time: 5 minutes

Serving Size: 1

Ingredients:

- 4 oz fresh tuna steak

- 1 tablespoon sesame seeds

- 2 cups mixed salad greens

- 1/4 cup cherry tomatoes, halved

- 1/4 cup cucumber, sliced

- 2 tablespoons low-sodium soy sauce

- 1 tablespoon rice vinegar

- 1 teaspoon sesame oil

Instructions:

1. Coat tuna steak with sesame seeds.

2. Heat a non-stick skillet over medium-high heat.

3. Sear tuna for 2-3 minutes on each side or until desired doneness.

4. In a bowl, whisk together soy sauce, rice vinegar, and sesame oil for the dressing.

5. Toss salad greens, cherry tomatoes, and cucumber with the sesame dressing.

6. Slice tuna and serve over the salad.

Nutritional Information:

- Calories: 330

- Protein: 25g

- Fiber: 4g

- Potassium: 320mg

- Phosphorus: 200mg

19. Black Bean and Vegetable Quesadilla

Prep Time: 15 minutes

Cooking Time: 10 minutes

Serving Size: 1

Ingredients:

- 1 whole-grain tortilla

- 1/2 cup black beans, cooked

- 1/4 cup bell peppers, diced

- 1/4 cup red onion, diced

- 1/4 cup low-fat shredded cheddar cheese

- 1 tablespoon fresh cilantro, chopped

Instructions:

1. Place tortilla on a griddle over medium heat.

2. Spread black beans, bell peppers, red onion, and cheddar cheese on one half of the tortilla.

3. Fold the tortilla in half and press with a spatula.

4. Cook for 4-5 minutes on each side or until cheese is melted and tortilla is golden brown.

5. Sprinkle with fresh cilantro before serving.

Nutritional Information:

- Calories: 310

- Protein: 18g

- Fiber: 8g

- Potassium: 280mg

- Phosphorus: 150mg

20. Zucchini Noodles with Pesto and Cherry Tomatoes

Prep Time: 15 minutes
Cooking Time: 5 minutes
Serving Size: 1

Ingredients:

- 1 medium zucchini, spiralized

- 1/2 cup cherry tomatoes, halved

- 2 tablespoons pesto sauce

- 1 tablespoon pine nuts, toasted

- Fresh basil leaves for garnish

Instructions:

1. In a skillet, sauté spiralized zucchini for 2-3 minutes until just tender.

2. Toss in cherry tomatoes and cook for an additional 1-2 minutes.

3. Stir in pesto sauce until well combined.

4. Transfer to a plate and sprinkle with toasted pine nuts and fresh basil leaves.

5. Serve immediately.

Nutritional Information:

- Calories: 290

- Protein: 8g

- Fiber: 4g

- Potassium: 350mg

- Phosphorus: 180mg

DINNER RECIPES

1. Grilled Lemon Herb Salmon

Prep Time: 15 minutes

Cooking Time: 15 minutes

Serving Size: 1

Ingredients:

- 4 oz salmon fillet

- 1 tablespoon olive oil

- 1 tablespoon lemon juice

- 1 teaspoon dried dill

- Salt and pepper to taste

Instructions:

1. Preheat the grill to medium-high heat.

2. Mix olive oil, lemon juice, dried dill, salt, and pepper in a bowl.

3. Brush the salmon fillet with the mixture.

4. Grill for 7-8 minutes per side or until salmon flakes easily.

5. Serve hot.

Nutritional Information:

- Calories: 320

- Protein: 25g

- Fiber: 0g

- Potassium: 400mg

- Phosphorus: 180mg

2. Chicken and Vegetable Kebabs

Prep Time: 20 minutes

Cooking Time: 15 minutes

Serving Size: 1

Ingredients:

- 4 oz chicken breast, cut into cubes

- Cherry tomatoes

- Bell peppers, sliced

- Red onion, cut into chunks

- Zucchini, sliced

- Olive oil

- Dried rosemary

- Salt and pepper to taste

Instructions:

1. Preheat the grill to medium-high heat.

2. Thread chicken and vegetables onto skewers.

3. Brush with olive oil, sprinkle with dried rosemary, salt, and pepper.

4. Grill for 10-12 minutes, turning occasionally.

5. Serve hot.

Nutritional Information:

- Calories: 280

- Protein: 30g

- Fiber: 4g

- Potassium: 350mg

- Phosphorus: 200mg

3. Shrimp and Quinoa Stir-Fry

Prep Time: 15 minutes

Cooking Time: 15 minutes

Serving Size: 1

Ingredients:

- 4 oz shrimp, peeled and deveined

- 1/2 cup cooked quinoa

- Broccoli florets

- Carrots, sliced

- Snap peas

- Low-sodium soy sauce

- Sesame oil

- Garlic, minced

Instructions:

1. In a wok or skillet, heat sesame oil over medium-high heat.

2. Add shrimp, broccoli, carrots, and snap peas. Stir-fry for 5-7 minutes.

3. Add cooked quinoa and minced garlic. Mix well.

4. Pour low-sodium soy sauce over the mixture and cook for an additional 2-3 minutes.

5. Serve hot.

Nutritional Information:

- Calories: 290

- Protein: 25g

- Fiber: 6g

- Potassium: 320mg

- Phosphorus: 180mg

4. Baked Lemon Herb Chicken

Prep Time: 15 minutes

Cooking Time: 25 minutes

Serving Size: 1

Ingredients:

- 4 oz chicken breast

- 1 tablespoon olive oil

- 1 tablespoon lemon juice

- Dried thyme

- Garlic powder

- Salt and pepper to taste

Instructions:

1. Preheat the oven to 400°F (200°C).

2. Place the chicken breast on a baking sheet.

3. Mix olive oil, lemon juice, dried thyme, garlic powder, salt, and pepper in a bowl.

4. Brush the chicken with the mixture.

5. Bake for 20-25 minutes or until the chicken is cooked through.

6. Serve hot.

Nutritional Information:

- Calories: 300

- Protein: 30g

- Fiber: 0g

- Potassium: 350mg

- Phosphorus: 200mg

5. Eggplant Parmesan

Prep Time: 20 minutes

Cooking Time: 30 minutes

Serving Size: 1

Ingredients:

- 1 small eggplant, sliced

- 1 cup marinara sauce (low-sodium)

- 1/2 cup low-fat mozzarella cheese, shredded

- 2 tablespoons Parmesan cheese, grated

- Fresh basil leaves for garnish

Instructions:

1. Preheat the oven to 375°F (190°C).

2. Arrange eggplant slices on a baking sheet.

3. Spoon marinara sauce over each slice.

4. Sprinkle with mozzarella and Parmesan cheese.

5. Bake for 25-30 minutes or until the cheese is bubbly and golden.

6. Garnish with fresh basil leaves and serve.

Nutritional Information:

- Calories: 290

- Protein: 15g

- Fiber: 8g

- Potassium: 400mg

- Phosphorus: 180mg

6. Turkey and Vegetable Skillet

Prep Time: 15 minutes
Cooking Time: 20 minutes
Serving Size: 1

Ingredients:

- 4 oz ground turkey

- Bell peppers, sliced

- Zucchini, sliced

- Red onion, sliced

- Olive oil

- Taco seasoning

- Black beans, cooked

- Low-fat Greek yogurt (optional)

Instructions:

1. In a skillet, heat olive oil over medium heat.

2. Add ground turkey and cook until browned.

3. Add sliced bell peppers, zucchini, and red onion. Sauté until vegetables are tender.

4. Stir in taco seasoning and cooked black beans.

5. Cook for an additional 5 minutes.

6. Serve hot with a dollop of low-fat Greek yogurt if desired.

Nutritional Information:

- Calories: 320

- Protein: 25g

- Fiber: 8g

- Potassium: 350mg

- Phosphorus: 200mg

7. Seared Tofu with Vegetable Medley

Prep Time: 20 minutes

Cooking Time: 15 minutes

Serving Size: 1

Ingredients:

- 1/2 cup firm tofu, cubed

- Broccoli florets

- Carrots, sliced

- Snow peas

- Low-sodium soy sauce

- Sesame oil

- Ginger, minced

- Brown rice (optional)

Instructions:

1. In a wok or skillet, heat sesame oil over medium-high heat.

2. Add cubed tofu, broccoli, carrots, and snow peas. Stir-fry for 8-10 minutes.

3. Mix in minced ginger and low-sodium soy sauce.

4. Cook for an additional 2-3 minutes.

5. Serve over brown rice if desired.

Nutritional Information:

- Calories: 280

- Protein: 15g

- Fiber: 7g

- Potassium: 320mg

- Phosphorus: 180mg

8. Lemon Garlic Shrimp Pasta

Prep Time: 15 minutes

Cooking Time: 20 minutes

Serving Size: 1

Ingredients:

- 2 oz whole-grain spaghetti

- 4 oz shrimp, peeled and deveined

- 1 tablespoon olive oil

- 1 tablespoon lemon juice

- Garlic, minced

- Cherry tomatoes, halved

- Spinach leaves

Instructions:

1. Cook pasta according to package instructions.

2. In a skillet, heat olive oil over medium heat.

3. Add shrimp and minced garlic. Cook for 2-3 minutes.

4. Stir in cherry tomatoes, spinach, and lemon juice.

5. Continue cooking until shrimp are opaque and vegetables are tender.

6. Toss with cooked spaghetti and serve.

Nutritional Information:

- Calories: 330

- Protein: 25g

- Fiber: 6g

- Potassium: 350mg

- Phosphorus: 200mg

9. Roasted Vegetable and Chickpea Salad

Prep Time: 20 minutes

Cooking Time: 25 minutes

Serving Size: 1

Ingredients:

- 1 cup cauliflower florets

- 1 cup sweet potato, diced

- 1 cup cherry tomatoes, halved

- 1/2 cup red onion, sliced

- 1/2 cup canned chickpeas, drained and rinsed

- Olive oil

- Dried rosemary

- Balsamic vinegar

- Feta cheese, crumbled (optional)

Instructions:

1. Preheat the oven to 400°F (200°C).

2. Toss cauliflower, sweet potato, cherry tomatoes, red onion, and chickpeas with olive oil and dried rosemary.

3. Roast for 20-25 minutes or until vegetables are tender.

4. Drizzle with balsamic vinegar and toss.

5. Sprinkle with crumbled feta cheese if desired.

Nutritional Information:

- Calories: 290

- Protein: 12g

- Fiber: 8g

- Potassium: 350mg

- Phosphorus: 180mg

10. Mediterranean Stuffed Bell Peppers

Prep Time: 20 minutes

Cooking Time: 30 minutes

Serving Size: 1

Ingredients:

- Bell peppers, halved and seeds removed

- 4 oz ground turkey

- Quinoa, cooked

- Cherry tomatoes, diced

- Kalamata olives, chopped

- Feta cheese, crumbled

- Olive oil

- Dried oregano

Instructions:

1. Preheat the oven to 375°F (190°C).

2. In a skillet, cook ground turkey until browned.

3. In a bowl, mix cooked quinoa, diced cherry tomatoes, chopped Kalamata olives, and crumbled feta cheese.

4. Stuff bell peppers with the quinoa mixture and cooked ground turkey.

5. Drizzle with olive oil and sprinkle with dried oregano.

6. Bake for 25-30 minutes or until peppers are tender.

Nutritional Information:

- Calories: 310

- Protein: 20g

- Fiber: 5g

- Potassium: 380mg

- Phosphorus: 200mg

11. Teriyaki Salmon with Broccoli

Prep Time: 15 minutes

Cooking Time: 20 minutes

Serving Size: 1

Ingredients:

- 4 oz salmon fillct

- Broccoli florets

- Low-sodium teriyaki sauce

- Garlic powder

- Sesame seeds for garnish

Instructions:

1. Preheat the oven to 400°F (200°C).

2. Place salmon on a baking sheet and surround with broccoli florets.

3. Brush salmon with low-sodium teriyaki sauce and sprinkle with garlic powder.

4. Bake for 15-20 minutes or until salmon is cooked through.

5. Garnish with sesame seeds and serve.

Nutritional Information:

- Calories: 320

- Protein: 25g

- Fiber: 0g

- Potassium: 400mg

- Phosphorus: 180mg

12. Lentil and Vegetable Stuffed Peppers

Prep Time: 20 minutes

Cooking Time: 30 minutes

Serving Size: 1

Ingredients:

- Bell peppers, halved and seeds removed

- 1/2 cup dried green lentils, rinsed

- Carrots, diced

- Celery, diced

- Onion, chopped

- Low-sodium vegetable broth

- Dried thyme

- Tomato sauce

Instructions:

1. Preheat the oven to 375°F (190°C).

2. Cook lentils in vegetable broth with carrots, celery, and onion until tender.

3. Mix in dried thyme and tomato sauce.

4. Stuff bell peppers with the lentil and vegetable mixture.

5. Bake for 25-30 minutes or until peppers are soft.

Nutritional Information:

- Calories: 280

- Protein: 18g

- Fiber: 10g

- Potassium: 400mg

- Phosphorus: 200mg

13. Spinach and Mushroom Stuffed Chicken Breast

Prep Time: 20 minutes

Cooking Time: 25 minutes

Serving Size: 1

Ingredients:

- 4 oz chicken breast

- Spinach, chopped

- Mushrooms, sliced

- Low-fat mozzarella cheese, shredded

- Olive oil

- Garlic powder

- Paprika

Instructions:

1. Preheat the oven to 375°F (190°C).

2. Butterfly the chicken breast and pound to an even thickness.

3. Sauté spinach and mushrooms in olive oil until wilted.

4. Spread the spinach and mushroom mixture on one half of the chicken breast.

5. Sprinkle with shredded mozzarella, garlic powder, and paprika.

6. Fold the other half of the chicken breast over the filling.

7. Bake for 20-25 minutes or until chicken is cooked through.

Nutritional Information:

- Calories: 300

- Protein: 30g

- Fiber: 2g

- Potassium: 350mg

- Phosphorus: 200mg

14. Cauliflower and Chickpea Stir-Fry

Prep Time: 15 minutes

Cooking Time: 20 minutes

Serving Size: 1

Ingredients:

- 1 cup cauliflower florets

- 1/2 cup canned chickpeas, drained and rinsed

- Carrots, sliced

- Snap peas

- Low-sodium soy sauce

- Sesame oil

- Ginger, minced

- Brown rice (optional)

Instructions:

1. In a wok or skillet, heat sesame oil over medium-high heat.

2. Add cauliflower, chickpeas, carrots, and snap peas. Stir-fry for 8-10 minutes.

3. Mix in minced ginger and low-sodium soy sauce.

4. Cook for an additional 2-3 minutes.

5. Serve over brown rice if desired.

Nutritional Information:

- Calories: 280

- Protein: 15g

- Fiber: 7g

- Potassium: 320mg

- Phosphorus: 180mg

15. Quinoa and Black Bean Stuffed Acorn Squash

Prep Time: 20 minutes

Cooking Time: 40 minutes

Serving Size: 1

Ingredients:

- 1 acorn squash, halved and seeds removed

- 1/2 cup cooked quinoa

- 1/2 cup black beans, cooked

- Red bell pepper, diced

- Red onion, diced

- Cumin

- Chili powder

- Fresh cilantro for garnish

Instructions:

1. Preheat the oven to 400°F (200°C).

2. Place acorn squash halves on a baking sheet.

3. In a bowl, mix cooked quinoa, black beans, red bell pepper, and red onion.

4. Season with cumin and chili powder.

5. Stuff each acorn squash half with the quinoa mixture.

6. Bake for 35-40 minutes or until squash is tender.

7. Garnish with fresh cilantro and serve.

Nutritional Information:

- Calories: 290

- Protein: 12g

- Fiber: 8g

- Potassium: 350mg

- Phosphorus: 180mg

16. Tomato Basil Chicken Pasta

Prep Time: 15 minutes

Cooking Time: 20 minutes

Serving Size: 1

Ingredients:

- 2 oz whole-grain penne pasta

- 4 oz chicken breast, diced

- Cherry tomatoes, halved

- Fresh basil leaves, chopped

- Olive oil

- Garlic, minced

- Salt and pepper to taste

Instructions:

1. Cook pasta according to package instructions.

2. In a skillet, heat olive oil over medium heat.

3. Add diced chicken and minced garlic. Cook for 5-7 minutes.

4. Stir in cherry tomatoes and cook until they start to soften.

5. Toss cooked pasta with the chicken and tomato mixture.

6. Season with salt, pepper, and fresh basil.

7. Serve hot.

Nutritional Information:

- Calories: 330

- Protein: 25g

- Fiber: 6g

- Potassium: 350mg

- Phosphorus: 200mg

17. Sweet Potato and Turkey Chili

Prep Time: 20 minutes

Cooking Time: 30 minutes

Serving Size: 1

Ingredients:

- 4 oz ground turkey

- Sweet potato, diced

- Black beans, cooked

- Diced tomatoes

- Low-sodium vegetable broth

- Chili powder

- Cumin

- Paprika

Instructions:

1. In a pot, brown ground turkey over medium heat.

2. Add diced sweet potato, black beans, diced tomatoes, and vegetable broth.

3. Season with chili powder, cumin, and paprika.

4. Simmer for 20-25 minutes or until sweet potatoes are tender.

5. Serve hot.

Nutritional Information:

- Calories: 310

- Protein: 20g

- Fiber: 8g

- Potassium: 380mg

- Phosphorus: 200mg

18. Grilled Vegetable and Quinoa Salad

Prep Time: 15 minutes

Cooking Time: 15 minutes

Serving Size: 1

Ingredients:

- 1/2 cup cooked quinoa

- Zucchini, sliced

- Cherry tomatoes, halved

- Red bell pepper, sliced

- Red onion, sliced

- Olive oil

- Balsamic vinegar

- Fresh parsley for garnish

Instructions:

1. Cook quinoa according to package instructions.

2. Preheat the grill to medium-high heat.

3. Grill zucchini, cherry tomatoes, red bell pepper, and red onion until lightly charred.

4. In a bowl, mix cooked quinoa and grilled vegetables.

5. Drizzle with olive oil and balsamic vinegar. Toss gently.

6. Garnish with fresh parsley and serve.

Nutritional Information:

- Calories: 280

- Protein: 10g

- Fiber: 7g

- Potassium: 350mg

- Phosphorus: 180mg

19. Baked Cod with Lemon and Herbs

Prep Time: 15 minutes

Cooking Time: 20 minutes

Serving Size: 1

Ingredients:

- 4 oz cod fillet

- Lemon slices

- Fresh dill, chopped

- Garlic powder

- Olive oil

- Salt and pepper to taste

Instructions:

1. Preheat the oven to 400°F (200°C).

2. Place cod fillet on a baking sheet.

3. Drizzle with olive oil and sprinkle with garlic powder, salt, and pepper.

4. Top with lemon slices and fresh dill.

5. Bake for 15-20 minutes or until the fish flakes easily.

6. Serve hot.

Nutritional Information:

- Calories: 310

- Protein: 30g

- Fiber: 0g

- Potassium: 350mg

- Phosphorus: 180mg

20. Stuffed Portobello Mushrooms

Prep Time: 20 minutes

Cooking Time: 25 minutes

Serving Size: 1

Ingredients:

- Portobello mushrooms, stems removed

- 1/2 cup quinoa, cooked

- Spinach, chopped

- Feta cheese, crumbled

- Cherry tomatoes, diced

- Balsamic glaze for drizzling

Instructions:

1. Preheat the oven to 375°F (190°C).

2. Place Portobello mushrooms on a baking sheet.

3. In a bowl, mix cooked quinoa, chopped spinach, crumbled feta, and diced cherry tomatoes.

4. Stuff each mushroom with the quinoa mixture.

5. Bake for 20-25 minutes or until mushrooms are tender.

6. Drizzle with balsamic glaze before serving.

Nutritional Information:

- Calories: 290

- Protein: 15g

- Fiber: 8g

- Potassium: 380mg

- Phosphorus: 200mg

DESSERT RECIPES

1. Berry Parfait

Prep Time: 15 minutes

Cooking Time: 0 minutes

Serving Size: 1

Ingredients:

- 1/2 cup low-fat Greek yogurt

- 1/4 cup mixed berries (blueberries, strawberries, raspberries)

- 1 tablespoon honey

- 1 tablespoon chopped nuts (almonds or walnuts)

Instructions:

1. In a glass, layer Greek yogurt, mixed berries, and chopped nuts.

2. Drizzle honey over the top.

3. Repeat the layers.

4. Serve chilled.

Nutritional Information:

- Calories: 150

- Protein: 10g

- Fiber: 3g

- Potassium: 200mg

- Phosphorus: 100mg

2. Baked Apples with Cinnamon

Prep Time: 10 minutes

Cooking Time: 30 minutes

Serving Size: 1

Ingredients:

- 1 medium apple, cored and halved

- 1/2 teaspoon cinnamon

- 1 tablespoon chopped nuts (pecans or almonds)

- 1 teaspoon honey

Instructions:

1. Preheat the oven to 375°F (190°C).

2. Place apple halves on a baking sheet.

3. Sprinkle with cinnamon and chopped nuts.

4. Drizzle honey over the top.

5. Bake for 25-30 minutes or until apples are tender.

6. Serve warm.

Nutritional Information:

- Calories: 120

- Protein: 2g

- Fiber: 4g

- Potassium: 180mg

- Phosphorus: 60mg

3. Mango Sorbet

Prep Time: 10 minutes

Cooking Time: 0 minutes

Serving Size: 1

Ingredients:

- 1 cup frozen mango chunks

- 1/4 cup coconut water

- 1 tablespoon lime juice

- Fresh mint leaves for garnish

Instructions:

1. In a blender, combine frozen mango chunks, coconut water, and lime juice.

2. Blend until smooth.

3. Scoop into a bowl and garnish with fresh mint leaves.

4. Serve immediately.

Nutritional Information:

- Calories: 100

- Protein: 1g

- Fiber: 2g

- Potassium: 150mg

- Phosphorus: 30mg

4. Chia Seed Pudding

Prep Time: 5 minutes (plus overnight chilling)

Cooking Time: 0 minutes

Serving Size: 1

Ingredients:

- 2 tablespoons chia seeds

- 1/2 cup unsweetened almond milk

- 1/4 teaspoon vanilla extract

- 1 tablespoon sliced strawberries

- 1 tablespoon blueberries

Instructions:

1. In a bowl, mix chia seeds, almond milk, and vanilla extract.

2. Stir well and refrigerate overnight.

3. Before serving, top with sliced strawberries and blueberries.

4. Stir gently and enjoy.

Nutritional Information:

- Calories: 120

- Protein: 4g

- Fiber: 8g

- Potassium: 120mg

- Phosphorus: 80mg

5. Almond Flour Cookies

Prep Time: 15 minutes

Cooking Time: 12 minutes

Serving Size: 2 cookies

Ingredients:

- 1 cup almond flour

- 1/4 cup unsalted butter, softened

- 2 tablespoons honey

- 1/2 teaspoon vanilla extract

- 1/4 cup dark chocolate chips

Instructions:

1. Preheat the oven to 350°F (180°C).

2. In a bowl, mix almond flour, softened butter, honey, and vanilla extract.

3. Fold in dark chocolate chips.

4. Drop spoonfuls of dough onto a baking sheet.

5. Bake for 10-12 minutes or until edges are golden.

6. Allow to cool before serving.

Nutritional Information:

- Calories: 180

- Protein: 4g

- Fiber: 2g

- Potassium: 50mg

- Phosphorus: 60mg

6. Watermelon Mint Salad

Prep Time: 10 minutes

Cooking Time: 0 minutes

Serving Size: 1

Ingredients:

- 1 cup diced watermelon

- Fresh mint leaves, chopped

- 1 tablespoon lime juice

- 1 tablespoon crumbled feta cheese (optional)

Instructions:

1. In a bowl, combine diced watermelon and chopped mint.

2. Drizzle with lime juice and toss gently.

3. Top with crumbled feta cheese if desired.

4. Serve chilled.

Nutritional Information:

- Calories: 60

- Protein: 1g

- Fiber: 1g

- Potassium: 100mg

- Phosphorus: 20mg

7. Avocado Chocolate Mousse

Prep Time: 10 minutes

Cooking Time: 0 minutes

Serving Size: 1

Ingredients:

- 1 ripe avocado

- 2 tablespoons unsweetened cocoa powder

- 2 tablespoons honey

- 1/2 teaspoon vanilla extract

- Fresh berries for garnish

Instructions:

1. In a blender, combine ripe avocado, cocoa powder, honey, and vanilla extract.

2. Blend until smooth.

3. Scoop into a bowl and garnish with fresh berries.

4. Serve immediately.

Nutritional Information:

- Calories: 220

- Protein: 3g

- Fiber: 7g

- Potassium: 350mg

- Phosphorus: 60mg

8. Coconut Rice Pudding

Prep Time: 10 minutes

Cooking Time: 25 minutes

Serving Size: 1

Ingredients:

- 1/4 cup Arborio rice

- 1 cup coconut milk

- 2 tablespoons honey

- 1/4 teaspoon ground cinnamon

- 1/4 cup toasted coconut flakes

Instructions:

1. In a saucepan, combine Arborio rice and coconut milk.

2. Bring to a simmer and cook for 20-25 minutes, stirring occasionally.

3. Stir in honey and ground cinnamon.

4. Spoon into a bowl and top with toasted coconut flakes.

5. Serve warm.

Nutritional Information:

- Calories: 280

- Protein: 3g

- Fiber: 1g

- Potassium: 120mg

- Phosphorus: 40mg

9. Peach and Blueberry Compote

Prep Time: 10 minutes

Cooking Time: 15 minutes

Serving Size: 1

Ingredients:

- 1 peach, peeled and diced

- 1/4 cup blueberries

- 1 tablespoon honey

- 1/4 teaspoon cinnamon

- 1 tablespoon chopped almonds

Instructions:

1. In a saucepan, combine diced peach and blueberries.

2. Add honey and cinnamon, then simmer for 10-15 minutes.

3. Spoon the compote into a bowl and sprinkle with chopped almonds.

4. Serve warm.

Nutritional Information:

- Calories: 120

- Protein: 2g

- Fiber: 3g

- Potassium: 160mg

- Phosphorus: 30mg

10. Frozen Banana Bites

Prep Time: 10 minutes

Cooking Time: 0 minutes

Serving Size: 2

Ingredients:

- 1 banana, sliced

- 2 tablespoons almond butter

- 2 tablespoons shredded coconut

Instructions:

1. Spread almond butter on banana slices.

2. Sandwich two slices together to create banana bites.

3. Roll the edges in shredded coconut.

4. Place on a tray and freeze for at least 2 hours.

5. Serve frozen.

Nutritional Information:

- Calories: 150

- Protein: 3g

- Fiber: 4g

- Potassium: 220mg

- Phosphorus: 40mg

SNACKS RECIPES

1. Apple and Almond Butter Stack

Prep Time: 5 minutes

Cooking Time: 0 minutes

Serving Size: 1

Ingredients:

- 1 medium apple, sliced

- 2 tablespoons almond butter

Instructions:

1. Arrange apple slices on a plate.

2. Spread almond butter on each apple slice.

3. Stack them together.

4. Enjoy this quick and nutritious snack.

Nutritional Information:

- Calories: 150

- Protein: 4g

- Fiber: 4g

- Potassium: 200mg

- Phosphorus: 60mg

2. Greek Yogurt Parfait

Prep Time: 10 minutes

Cooking Time: 0 minutes

Serving Size: 1

Ingredients:

- 1/2 cup low-fat Greek yogurt

- 1/4 cup granola (low-phosphorus)

- 1/4 cup mixed berries (blueberries, strawberries)

- 1 tablespoon honey

Instructions:

1. In a glass, layer Greek yogurt, granola, and mixed berries.

2. Drizzle honey over the top.

3. Repeat the layers.

4. A delightful and protein-packed snack.

Nutritional Information:

- Calories: 200

- Protein: 10g

- Fiber: 3g

- Potassium: 250mg

- Phosphorus: 80mg

3. Cucumber and Hummus Bites

Prep Time: 10 minutes

Cooking Time: 0 minutes

Serving Size: 1

Ingredients:

- 1 medium cucumber, sliced

- 2 tablespoons hummus

Instructions:

1. Arrange cucumber slices on a plate.

2. Spoon a dollop of hummus on each slice.

3. A refreshing and low-calorie snack option.

Nutritional Information:

- Calories: 50

- Protein: 2g

- Fiber: 1g

- Potassium: 150mg

- Phosphorus: 40mg

4. Rice Cake with Cottage Cheese and Pineapple

Prep Time: 5 minutes

Cooking Time: 0 minutes

Serving Size: 1

Ingredients:

- 1 rice cake

- 1/2 cup low-fat cottage cheese

- 1/4 cup pineapple chunks (fresh or canned)

Instructions:

1. Spread cottage cheese on the rice cake.

2. Top with pineapple chunks.

3. A simple and satisfying low-sodium snack.

Nutritional Information:

- Calories: 120

- Protein: 10g

- Fiber: 1g

- Potassium: 150mg

- Phosphorus: 80mg

5. Hard-Boiled Egg and Cherry Tomatoes

Prep Time: 15 minutes

Cooking Time: 10 minutes

Serving Size: 1

Ingredients:

- 1 hard-boiled egg

- 1/2 cup cherry tomatoes

- Pinch of salt and pepper

Instructions:

1. Peel and slice the hard-boiled egg.

2. Arrange egg slices and cherry tomatoes on a plate.

3. Sprinkle with a pinch of salt and pepper.

4. A protein-rich and wholesome snack.

Nutritional Information:

- Calories: 130

- Protein: 10g

- Fiber: 2g

- Potassium: 200mg

- Phosphorus: 150mg

6. Trail Mix with Nuts and Dried Fruits

Prep Time: 5 minutes

Cooking Time: 0 minutes

Serving Size: 1

Ingredients:

- 1/4 cup mixed nuts (almonds, walnuts)

- 1 tablespoon dried cranberries

- 1 tablespoon raisins

Instructions:

1. Combine mixed nuts, dried cranberries, and raisins in a bowl.

2. Toss well and portion out.

3. A convenient and energy-boosting snack.

Nutritional Information:

- Calories: 180

- Protein: 5g

- Fiber: 3g

- Potassium: 200mg

- Phosphorus: 80mg

7. Cottage Cheese and Pineapple Skewers

Prep Time: 10 minutes

Cooking Time: 0 minutes

Serving Size: 1

Ingredients:

- 1/2 cup low-fat cottage cheese

- 1/2 cup pineapple chunks (fresh or canned)

- Skewers

Instructions:

1. Thread cottage cheese and pineapple chunks onto skewers.

2. Serve as a delightful and protein-rich snack.

Nutritional Information:

- Calories: 120

- Protein: 10g

- Fiber: 1g

- Potassium: 150mg

- Phosphorus: 80mg

8. Baked Sweet Potato Fries

Prep Time: 15 minutes

Cooking Time: 25 minutes

Serving Size: 1

Ingredients:

- 1 small sweet potato, cut into fries

- 1 tablespoon olive oil

- Pinch of salt and pepper

Instructions:

1. Preheat the oven to 425°F (220°C).

2. Toss sweet potato fries in olive oil, salt, and pepper.

3. Spread on a baking sheet and bake for 20-25 minutes.

4. A nutrient-packed alternative to traditional fries.

Nutritional Information:

- Calories: 120

- Protein: 2g

- Fiber: 3g

- Potassium: 220mg

- Phosphorus: 40mg

9. Sliced Bell Peppers with Guacamole

Prep Time: 10 minutes

Cooking Time: 0 minutes

Serving Size: 1

Ingredients:

- 1 bell pepper, sliced

- 2 tablespoons guacamole

Instructions:

1. Arrange bell pepper slices on a plate.

2. Serve with guacamole for a flavorful and healthy snack.

Nutritional Information:

- Calories: 80

- Protein: 2g

- Fiber: 3g

- Potassium: 250mg

- Phosphorus: 60mg

10. Edamame Beans with Sea Salt

Prep Time: 5 minutes

Cooking Time: 5 minutes

Serving Size: 1

Ingredients:

- 1/2 cup edamame beans (shelled)

- Sea salt to taste

Instructions:

1. Boil or steam edamame beans until tender.

2. Sprinkle with sea salt and toss.

3. A protein-packed and savory snack.

Nutritional Information:

- Calories: 100

- Protein: 9g

- Fiber: 4g

- Potassium: 150mg

- Phosphorus: 80mg

LIFESTYLE AND KIDNEY HEALTH

Our lifestyle choices play a pivotal role in maintaining overall health, and when it comes to kidney health, certain aspects of our daily routines can significantly impact these vital organs. In this exploration of "Lifestyle and Kidney Health," we delve into two key components: the "Importance of Physical Activity" and "Stress Management and Kidney Wellness." By understanding the intricate connections between our lifestyle choices and kidney health, we empower ourselves to make informed decisions that contribute to the longevity and well-being of these essential organs.

Importance of Physical Activity

Physical activity is often celebrated for its role in cardiovascular health, weight management, and overall well-being. However, its influence on kidney health is equally profound. Regular exercise can be likened to a powerhouse that not only strengthens muscles and improves cardiovascular function but also significantly contributes to the maintenance of healthy kidneys.

The kidneys, responsible for filtering waste and excess fluids from the blood, benefit immensely from physical activity. When we engage in regular exercise, our cardiovascular system becomes more efficient, promoting better blood flow. This improved circulation allows the kidneys to effectively carry out their filtration process. Moreover, exercise contributes to the regulation of blood pressure, a critical factor in kidney health. By reducing stress on blood vessels, physical activity assists in preventing conditions like hypertension, which, if left uncontrolled, can lead to kidney damage over time.

Aerobic exercises, such as walking, jogging, or swimming, are particularly beneficial for kidney health. These activities elevate heart rate and breathing, enhancing cardiovascular fitness. As the heart pumps more blood with each beat, the kidneys receive a steady supply, ensuring optimal filtration. Strength training exercises, like weightlifting or resistance training, also play a role. They help maintain a healthy body weight and can contribute to the prevention of conditions like diabetes, which is a common cause of kidney disease.

It is important to note that moderation is key. While regular physical activity offers numerous benefits, excessive or intense exercise, especially without proper hydration, may lead to dehydration and potentially harm the kidneys. Thus, striking a balance and staying adequately hydrated during and after exercise is crucial for kidney health.

Incorporating physical activity into our daily lives is a proactive step toward preserving kidney function. A sedentary lifestyle, on the other hand, can contribute to the development of risk factors such as obesity and hypertension, which are detrimental to kidney health. Therefore, finding enjoyable and sustainable ways to stay active is not only an investment in our overall well-being but specifically in the health of these vital organs.

Stress Management and Kidney Wellness

In the hustle and bustle of daily life, stress has become an almost ubiquitous companion. From work pressures to personal challenges, the modern world presents a myriad of stressors that can significantly impact our health. Stress, when chronic and unmanaged, can pose a threat to various bodily systems, including the kidneys.

Understanding the connection between stress management and kidney wellness is a crucial aspect of holistic health. The intricate relationship between stress and kidney function is bidirectional. Chronic stress can contribute to the development or exacerbation of kidney disease, while pre-existing kidney issues can also induce stress as individuals grapple with the complexities of managing their health.

The physiological response to stress involves the activation of the body's "fight or flight" mechanism, releasing hormones such as cortisol and adrenaline. While this response is adaptive in acute situations, chronic activation can lead to prolonged elevation of these stress hormones, which may contribute to kidney damage over time. Elevated stress hormones can cause blood vessels to constrict, reducing blood flow to the kidneys and potentially impairing their function.

Additionally, stress-induced behaviors, such as poor dietary choices, inadequate sleep, and increased consumption of stimulants like caffeine or alcohol, can further exacerbate the risk of kidney damage. For example, a diet high in processed and unhealthy foods may contribute to conditions like diabetes and hypertension, both of which are leading causes of kidney disease.

Conversely, individuals with pre-existing kidney conditions may experience heightened stress levels due to the demands of managing a chronic health issue. The constant monitoring of dietary restrictions, medications, and medical appointments can take a toll on mental well-being. Stress management becomes a crucial component of their overall care to prevent the negative impact of stress on kidney function.

Various stress management techniques have shown promise in supporting kidney health. Mindfulness practices, such as meditation and deep breathing exercises, can help regulate the body's stress response. Engaging in hobbies, spending time in nature, and fostering social connections are also effective ways to alleviate stress. Adequate sleep and a well-balanced, kidney-friendly diet further contribute to stress reduction.

28-DAY MEAL PLAN

Day 1:

- **Breakfast:** Quinoa and Berry Breakfast Bowl

- **Lunch:** Chicken Salad with Mixed Greens

- **Dinner:** Grilled Chicken with Lemon and Rosemary

- **Snack:** Apple and Almond Butter Stack

Day 2:

- **Breakfast:** Oatmeal with Almond Butter and Banana

- **Lunch:** Quinoa and Black Bean Bowl

- **Dinner:** Baked Salmon with Dill and Lemon

- **Snack:** Greek Yogurt Parfait

Day 3:

- **Breakfast:** Greek Yogurt Parfait with Mixed Berries

- **Lunch:** Greek Chicken Wrap

- **Dinner:** Vegetable and Chickpea Curry

- **Snack:** Cucumber and Hummus Bites

Day 4:

- **Breakfast:** Spinach and Feta Omelette

- **Lunch:** Lentil Soup with Vegetables

- **Dinner:** Turkey and Vegetable Stir-Fry

- **Snack:** Rice Cake with Cottage Cheese and Pineapple

Day 5:

- **Breakfast:** Whole Grain Pancakes with Blueberries

- **Lunch:** Turkey and Avocado Lettuce Wraps

- **Dinner:** Quinoa-Stuffed Bell Peppers

- **Snack:** Hard-Boiled Egg and Cherry Tomatoes

Day 6:

- **Breakfast:** Avocado Toast with Poached Egg

- **Lunch:** Grilled Salmon Salad

- **Dinner:** Chicken and Vegetable Skewers

- **Snack:** Trail Mix with Nuts and Dried Fruits

Day 7:

- **Breakfast:** Chia Seed Pudding with Mango

- **Lunch:** Chickpea and Vegetable Stir-Fry

- **Dinner:** Shrimp and Asparagus Stir-Fry

- **Snack:** Cottage Cheese and Pineapple Skewers

Day 8:

- **Breakfast:** Sweet Potato Hash with Turkey Sausage

- **Lunch:** Caprese Sandwich with Whole Grain Bread

- **Dinner:** Baked Cod with Lemon and Herbs

- **Snack:** Baked Sweet Potato Fries

Day 9:

- **Breakfast:** Cottage Cheese and Pineapple Smoothie

- **Lunch:** Sweet Potato and Black Bean Quesadilla

- **Dinner:** Tomato Basil Chicken Pasta

- **Snack:** Sliced Bell Peppers with Guacamole

Day 10:

- **Breakfast:** Egg Muffins with Vegetables

- **Lunch:** Caesar Salad with Grilled Chicken

- **Dinner:** Sweet Potato and Turkey Chili

- **Snack:** Edamame Beans with Sea Salt

Day 11:

- **Breakfast:** Apple Cinnamon Overnight Oats

- **Lunch:** Tomato Basil Soup with Whole Wheat Croutons

- **Dinner:** Grilled Vegetable and Quinoa Salad

- **Snack:** Greek Yogurt Parfait

Day 12:

- **Breakfast:** Smoothie Bowl with Spinach and Berries

- **Lunch:** Tuna Salad Stuffed Bell Peppers

- **Dinner:** Stuffed Portobello Mushrooms

- **Snack:** Rice Cake with Cottage Cheese and Pineapple

Day 13:

- **Breakfast:** Banana Walnut Muffins

- **Lunch:** Veggie Wrap with Hummus

- **Dinner:** Baked Chicken Parmesan

- **Snack:** Hard-Boiled Egg and Cherry Tomatoes

Day 14:

- **Breakfast:** Veggie Breakfast Burrito

- **Lunch:** Shrimp and Quinoa Salad

- **Dinner:** Spinach and Feta Stuffed Chicken Breast

- **Snack:** Trail Mix with Nuts and Dried Fruits

Day 15:

- **Breakfast:** Almond Flour Pancakes with Strawberries

- **Lunch:** Turkey and Vegetable Skewers

- **Dinner:** Black Bean and Vegetable Burrito Bowl

- **Snack:** Baked Sweet Potato Fries

Day 16:

- **Breakfast:** Breakfast Quiche with Spinach and Feta

- **Lunch:** Mediterranean Quinoa Bowl

- **Dinner:** Roasted Veggie and Brown Rice Bowl

- **Snack:** Sliced Bell Peppers with Guacamole

Day 17:

- **Breakfast:** Smoked Salmon and Cream Cheese Bagel

- **Lunch:** Broccoli and Cheddar Stuffed Baked Potatoes

- **Dinner:** Teriyaki Salmon with Sesame Broccoli

- **Snack:** Edamame Beans with Sea Salt

Day 18:

- **Breakfast:** Breakfast Wrap with Turkey and Avocado

- **Lunch:** Asian Chicken Lettuce Wraps

- **Dinner:** Turkey Meatball and Zucchini Noodles

- **Snack:** Cottage Cheese and Pineapple Skewers

Day 19:

- **Breakfast:** Blueberry and Almond Baked Oatmeal

- **Lunch:** Spinach and Mushroom Frittata

- **Dinner:** Spaghetti Squash with Pesto and Cherry Tomatoes

- **Snack:** Greek Yogurt Parfait

Day 20:

- **Breakfast:** Green Smoothie with Kale and Pineapple

- **Lunch:** Brown Rice Bowl with Teriyaki Tofu

- **Dinner:** Quinoa and Black Bean Stuffed Peppers

- **Snack:** Baked Sweet Potato Fries

Day 21:

- **Breakfast:** Berry Parfait

- **Lunch:** Chicken Salad with Mixed Greens

- **Dinner:** Grilled Chicken with Lemon and Rosemary

- **Snack:** Apple and Almond Butter Stack

Day 22:

- **Breakfast:** Baked Apples with Cinnamon

- **Lunch:** Quinoa and Black Bean Bowl

- **Dinner:** Baked Salmon with Dill and Lemon

- **Snack:** Greek Yogurt Parfait

Day 23:

- **Breakfast:** Mango Sorbet

- **Lunch:** Greek Chicken Wrap

- **Dinner:** Vegetable and Chickpea Curry

- **Snack:** Cucumber and Hummus Bites

Day 24:

- **Breakfast:** Chia Seed Pudding

- **Lunch:** Lentil Soup with Vegetables

- **Dinner:** Turkey and Vegetable Stir-Fry

- **Snack:** Rice Cake with Cottage Cheese and Pineapple

Day 25:

- **Breakfast:** Almond Flour Cookies

- **Lunch:** Turkey and Avocado Lettuce Wraps

- **Dinner:** Quinoa-Stuffed Bell Peppers

- **Snack:** Hard-Boiled Egg and Cherry Tomatoes

Day 26:

- **Breakfast:** Watermelon Mint Salad

- **Lunch:** Grilled Salmon Salad

- **Dinner:** Chicken and Vegetable Skewers

- **Snack:** Trail Mix with Nuts and Dried Fruits

Day 27:

- **Breakfast:** Avocado Chocolate Mousse

- **Lunch:** Chickpea and Vegetable Stir-Fry

- **Dinner:** Shrimp and Asparagus Stir-Fry

- **Snack:** Cottage Cheese and Pineapple Skewers

Day 28:

- **Breakfast:** Coconut Rice Pudding

- **Lunch:** Caprese Sandwich with Whole Grain Bread

- **Dinner:** Baked Cod with Lemon and Herbs

- **Snack:** Baked Sweet Potato Fries

CONCLUSION

As we bring this culinary journey to a close within the pages of the "Stage 4 Kidney Disease Diet Cookbook for Seniors," it's not just about recipes but a heartfelt exploration into the symbiotic relationship between delicious food and kidney health.

In the realm of health, particularly for seniors grappling with Stage 4 Kidney Disease, the significance of a thoughtfully crafted diet cannot be overstated. This cookbook, more than a mere collection of recipes, has been a companion on the path toward nourishment that goes beyond sustenance—it's about embracing flavor, variety, and the sheer joy of a well-prepared meal.

The journey began with an understanding of the intricate dance our kidneys perform daily, filtering and regulating, silently contributing to our vitality. In "The Basics of Stage 4 Kidney Disease," we demystified the complexities, from an overview of kidney function to navigating the symptoms and challenges inherent in this stage. It was about knowledge—knowing our bodies, understanding the signals they send, and responding with care.

"The Senior Perspective" delved into the unique considerations of aging gracefully with kidney disease. It recognized the importance of managing kidney health alongside other health concerns, acknowledging the interconnected nature of our well-being. This section was a testament to resilience and adaptability, reminding us that every meal is a chance to nourish not just the body but the spirit.

In "The Kidney-Friendly Kitchen," we explored the heart of every home—the kitchen. Stocking a kidney-friendly pantry became a culinary adventure, and mastering essential cooking tools and techniques transformed the kitchen into a canvas for creativity. It wasn't just about following a diet; it was about embracing a lifestyle, where the act of cooking became an expression of self-care.

"Nutritional Guidelines for Seniors with Kidney Disease" provided a compass through the landscape of nutrient restrictions and offered practical tips for maintaining a balanced diet. It was a gentle reminder that, even in the face of limitations, the palette of possibilities remained vibrant and varied.

The recipes—oh, the recipes! From breakfast to dinner, and every snack in between, each dish was a celebration of flavors carefully curated to align with the dietary needs of those navigating Stage 4 Kidney Disease. The meal plans weren't just about sustenance; they were a testament to the richness of life that could be savored even within the constraints of a specialized diet.

As we bid adieu to these pages, let's not think of it as closing a book but rather savoring the last bite of a delicious meal. The "Stage 4 Kidney Disease Diet Cookbook for Seniors" isn't just a guide; it's a companion on a gastronomic journey towards well-being. It's about embracing the pleasure of eating while being mindful of the nourishment each bite brings.

So here's to health, to vibrant meals that dance on the taste buds, and to the wisdom that comes with understanding and caring for our bodies. May these recipes continue to grace kitchens, sparking joy in each preparation and adding a dash of flavor to the journey of those navigating Stage 4 Kidney Disease.